CaregiversAdvisors.org

Emergency Go-to-Guide

The Information You Need at Hand to Care for Your Parents or Grandparents

By: Jack Rosenberg, M.D.

Caregivers Advisors
1003 Willow Creek Road
Prescott, AZ 86301
www.CaregiversAdvisors.org

Copyright © 2013 by Jack Rosenberg, M.D.
All rights reserved. No part of this book may be copied, transmitted or stored in a database without permission.

DISCLAIMER

This book is not intended as medical advice. It is also not intended to prevent, diagnose, treat or cure disease. Instead the book is intended only to share the unofficial research and opinion of the author. The information is provided for educational purposes only, not as treatment instructions for any disease or ailment. Much of the book is a statement of opinion in areas where the facts are controversial or do not exist. The information in this book should not be considered any more valid than any other type of informal opinion.

The information was not written to replace the advice or care of a qualified health care professional. Be sure to check with your own qualified health care provider before beginning any protocols or procedures discussed in this book, or before stopping or altering any diet, lifestyle, or other therapies previously recommended to you by your health care provider.

The treatments described in this book may have side effects and carry other known and unknown risks and health hazards. The statements in this book have not been evaluated by the United States FDA. Use of the information in this book is at your own risk.

DEDICATION

This book is dedicated to Mrs. JoAnne Lerner, our loving mother, who currently lives with us, and suffers from severe dementia. She is loving, caring and never stops amazing us

A MESSAGE TO ALL SRUGLLING CAREGIVERS

Sometimes life turns around and the person who has taken care of you all your life starts to need care themselves. If your loved one is also dealing with degenerative diseases like Alzheimer's or dementia it's a big task not only for you but for the whole family as well.

I am Dr. Jack Rosenberg. My wife's mother is suffering from severe dementia and we have gone down the same road that you are walking on right now; facing the same heartbreaking decisions that you face. It is my purpose to empower you to make good decisions for your loved one's health using the knowledge and experience I've obtained as a medical doctor for the past 20+ years.

It was months of frustration for me to learn the ins and outs of all the documentation, legal forms and information that I needed to compile in order to get the treatment necessary for my mother-in-law. Finally, to alleviate the stress, I organized the whole mess into my Go-to-Packet. This is an essential guide I use to help my own mother-in-law and it will help alleviate the stress of caregiving for you too.

I hope that by downloading the Go-to-Packet you'll get organized to make caring for your loved ones a little easier. This packet is meant to be printed out and filled out. To get the printable version of the Go-to-Packet, just check my site: http://CaregiversAdvisors.org/print. For all your inquiries on caregiving, feel free to send me an email.

All the best,
Dr. Jack Rosenberg
drrosenberg@caregiversadvisors.org.

CONTENTS

Important Names and Phone Numbers 1

Medical Information: What to Tell 911 3

Authorization to Release Healthcare Information 5

Do Not Resuscitate Order 7

Driver's License Copy 8

Medical Insurance Card Copy 9

Medicare Supplement Card Copy 10

Recommended Reading 13

About the Author 17

Emergency Go-to-Guide

IMPORTANT NAMES AND PHONE NUMBERS

Cell Phone Number of Loved One (grandma/grandpa/mom/dad):
Home Number:
Emergency Contacts (Spouse, brothers, sisters)   Name: Complete Address: Contact Number: Pharmacy Phone Number: Physical Therapy Number and Address:
Indicate the names of doctor and phone number if you have more than one   Name of Doctor: Phone Number: Doctor's specialty: Name of Doctor:

Jack Rosenberg, M.D.

Phone Number:

Doctor's specialty:

Name of Doctor:

Phone Number:

Doctor's specialty:

Name of Doctor:

Phone Number:

Doctor's specialty:

Name of Doctor:

Phone Number:

Doctor's specialty:

MEDICAL INFORMATION: WHAT TO TELL 911

Allergies:

Medications:

Medicine:

Dosage/day:

Medicine:

Dosage/day:

Medicine:

Dosage/day:

Current Medical Conditions:

List of Supplements (herbal supplements, vitamins and other over the counter medications taken):

List of All past Surgeries:
Doctor's Name:
Phone Number:

Authorization to Release Healthcare Information

Patient's Name:
Date of Birth:
Previous Name:
Social Security #:
I request and authorize: To release healthcare information of the patient named above to: Name: Address: City: State: Zip Code:
This request and authorization applies to:
Healthcare information relating to the following treatment, condition, or dates:

All Healthcare Information:

Other:

☐ Yes   ☐ No

I authorize the release of any record regarding drug, alcohol, or mental health treatment to the person(s) listed above.

Patient Signature:

Date Signed:

THIS AUTHORIZATION EXPIRES NINETY DAYS AFTER IT IS SIGNED.

Emergency Go-to-Guide

Do Not Resuscitate Order

Click here to find out more about DO NOT Resuscitate Order and print one off for your state

If your loved one has a Do Not Resuscitate order, please include it here.

Keep any and all Copies of Paperwork attached to this packet at all times.

DRIVER'S LICENSE COPY

Make a copy of your parents' driver's license (front and back) and place it here:

MEDICAL INSURANCE CARD COPY

Make a copy of your patient's Medicare card (front and back) and place it here:

Jack Rosenberg, M.D.

MEDICARE SUPPLEMENT CARD COPY

Make a copy of the Medicare supplement card (front and back) and place it here:

Your Address:

Grandma and Grandpa's Address (if separate):

Jack Rosenberg, M.D.

RECOMMENDED READING

In researching for my own family, I found these to be helpful. You can check them out on my site here:

http://CaregiversAdvisors.org/Recommended

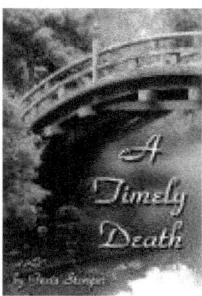

A Timely Death

A book that explores the meaningful relationship of a family, the damage that Alzheimer's brought, and the lengths that we are willing to reach for the ones we love.

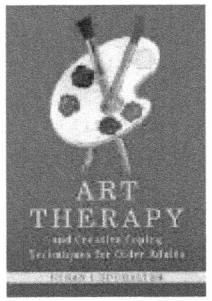

Art Therapy and Creative Coping Techniques for Older Adults

Suitable for older adults, including those with anxiety, depression or in the early stages of dementia, this will be an essential tool for art therapists as well as counselors, carers, psychotherapists, and social workers.

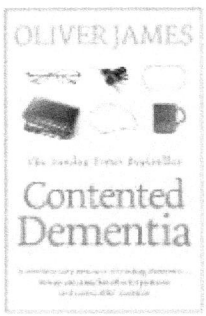

Contented Dementia: 24-hour Wraparound Care for Lifelong Well-being

A Dementia patient will usually experience random and frequently increased memory blanks to recent events. However, their feelings remain the same and the memories of past events are intact. Both of these can be utilize in a special way to replace for the recent information that has been lost. The SPECAL method (Specialized Early Care for Alzheimer's) outlined in this book works by creating links between past memories and the routine activities of daily life in the present.

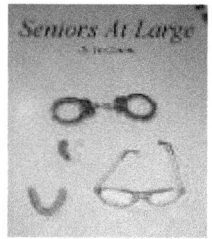

Seniors At Large

Eight elderly patients escaped their nursing home due to mistreatment. They had a hilarious, fun filled adventure, before ultimately redeeming themselves.

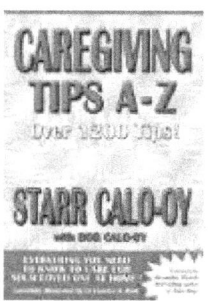

Caregiving Tips A-Z

All you need to know in providing care for your loved ones at home!

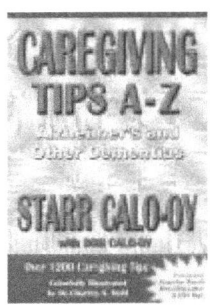

Caregiving Tips A-Z Alzheimer's & Other Dementias

All you need to know in providing care for your loved ones at home, especially the ones with Alzheimer's and Dementia.

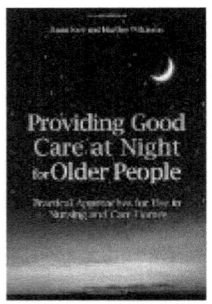

Providing Good Care at Night for Older People: Practical Approaches for Use in Nursing and Care Homes

This should be a good reference for night staff and their managers and employers, as well as inspectors of services, policy makers, and anyone else with an interest in the provision of care for older people.

ABOUT THE AUTHOR

Doctor Jack Rosenberg – Board Certified physician. Graduated high school in Phoenix, Arizona as a member of the class of 1981. He later attended college where he received his B.S, Bachelors of Science degree, in Biology at the University of Arizona. There he graduated with Suma Cum Laude, High Distinction and Honors as a 1986 graduate. He was also a member of the Phi Beta Kappa. A strong advocate for excellence and education, he involved himself with continuing education and hard work. Doctor Rosenberg attended Medical school at the Medical College of Wisconsin (Marquette University) and graduated in 1991. For his residency he worked at the William Beaumont Hospital in Royal Oak, Michigan specializing in Obstetrics and Gynecology finishing in 1995. His professional interests focus on the health of others, helping others, and hard work to better others which lead to him creating his own private practice in Prescott, Arizona since 1997.

Doctor Rosenberg has garnered many high achievements that have helped others in his community as well as better himself. Education is of high importance to him as proven through his hard work and dedication to his goals and choices in life. He has made himself as well as his family proud. He is a true leader to his community. He likes hiking, tennis, boating, and spending time with his family. In addition, he serves as the husband of his beautiful wife of 23 years Jennifer Rosenberg. He also serves as the father of two children Collin and Beverly. Jennifer's mother has dementia and has been living with the Rosenberg's for about a year. Dementia is a brain disorder that cause memory disorders such as Alzheimer's. Doctor and Mrs. Rosenberg dedicate their time, not only to their careers, but also to their family and friends. Doctor Jack Rosenberg is of great excellence promoting education, family, aid, and more.

You can find Dr. Rosenberg on Google+ and Facebook. It is his purpose to empower caregivers of aging relatives to make good decisions for their loved ones health.

Jack Rosenberg, M.D.

www.ingramcontent.com/pod-product-compliance
Lightning Source LLC
Chambersburg PA
CBHW070734180526
45167CB00004B/1756